WHAT IF IT'S ADHD and College: 25 Questions Answered

Skinny Book™

By:
Paul Nevin, PsyD
&
Kerri Nevin, PsyD

Copyright © 2012 Dr. Paul Nevin & Dr. Kerri Nevin

All rights reserved

ISBN: 978-0-9853555-3-1

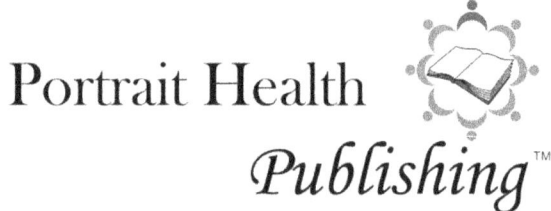

Published by Portrait Health Publishing, Inc.
2201 Waukegan Road, Suite 170, Bannockburn, IL 60015
www.portraithealthpublishing.com

Cover Design by Jeremy Shape

Disclaimer

No part of this book may be reproduced in any form or by any electronic or mechanical means including information storage and retrieval systems without permission in writing from the author. The only exception is by a reviewer who may quote short excerpts in a review.

All trademarks are the property of their respective owners.

About the Authors

Dr. Paul Nevin and Dr. Kerri Nevin are a husband and wife team of Clinical Psychologists who have been working with ADHD children, adolescents and adults for over 20 years. Dr. Paul Nevin holds a doctoral degree in Clinical Psychology and also has a Masters degree in Developmental Psychology. Dr. Kerri Nevin holds a doctoral degree in Clinical Psychology and is also a Mayo Clinic Certified Wellness Coach. Dr. Paul and Dr. Kerri own and operate Heart Light Psychological Services (www.HeartLightPS.com) which is located in Bannockburn, Illinois. Drs. Paul and Kerri have three boys, one of whom has been diagnosed with ADHD.

TABLE OF CONTENTS

INTRODUCTION 6

PART I: HOW TO FIND AN ADHD-FRIENDLY COLLEGE 10

    Question 1: What is an ADHD-friendly college? 10
    Question 2: What are "accommodations?" 11
    Question 3: How do special education services during grade school and high school differ from the kind of help that students receive in college? 12
    Question 4: If the law determines what kind of help is given, why are there differences from one college to another? 14
    Question 5: Are there basic categories that colleges fall into with regard to the kind of help that they offer? 15
    TABLE 1: CATEGORIES OF SERVICES PROVIDED BY COLLEGES 17
    Question 6: How do I find out which schools might have good programs for ADHD students? 19
    Question 7: Are there scholarships available to ADHD students? 19
    Question 8: If I find an "ADHD-friendly" college, will my child be okay? 20
    Question 9: Other than accommodations and services available, what other factors might make a college ADHD-friendly? 21
    Question 10: What else (besides college choice) will help an ADHD teen make a good transition to college? 26
    Question 11: Is a school that had good services for learning disabilities also a good school for an ADHD child? 29

PART II: WHEN, WHERE AND HOW TO CONTACT COLLEGES REGARDING ADHD 32

    Question 12: Whom do I contact at the college to talk about accommodations and services provided for students with ADHD? 32
    Question 13: When should I first make contact with the college disability office? 32
    Question 14: How much do the professionals at the disability office know about ADHD? 33
    Question 15: Can I use the fact that my child has and IEP in high school to prove that he or she needs accommodations in college? 33
    Question 16: Can I have a Psychiatrist or other professional working with my child write a letter in order to prove that he or she needs accommodations in college? 34
    Question 17: What is needed in order for a college student to be granted disability status based on ADHD so as to be allowed access to the modifications and services provided by the college? 34

Question 18: If my child says something about their ADHD during the application process, could that be used as a basis for not accepting them into the college? 37
Question 19: If my child seeks help for ADHD during college, will that information be available in the future to employers? 37
Question 20: What, if anything, should my child say about their disability during the application process? 37
Question 21: What questions should I ask the college to find out if the school is ADHD-friendly? 38
TABLE 2. QUESTIONS TO ASK AT THE COLLEGE 39

PART III: UNDERSTANDING ADHD AND ITS IMPACT ON THE COLLEGE EXPERIENCE.....44

Question 22: Don't people outgrow ADHD as they move into adulthood? 44
Question 23: I've heard that ADHD is not even a real disorder -- that it is just a way for drug companies and others to make money by convincing people that they have a "disorder" and then selling them a medication. Is this true? 46
Question 24: Doesn't focusing too much on ADHD hurt a young adult's confidence and self-esteem? 47
Question 25: What questions are not answered in this book? 49

OTHER BOOKS COMING SOON! 51

RESOURCES 52

WEBSITES 54

Introduction

"Beth, are you okay?" One of the advantages of being married for over twenty years is that Jim could tell when his wife was feeling overwhelmed just by the feel of the air in the room. He hoped it wasn't anything too serious. Beth was sitting quietly by herself in the study. The room was almost dark. It wasn't like her at all.

"Beth, honey, what's wrong?" Beth sighed deeply. "What's wrong? Oh, just everything, that's all." Jim knew better than to say anything at this point. He had to wait and let her start to get it out in her own way. "I've put in a call to the college counselor that Michael spoke with at school, and he still hasn't called me back. Then, while I was waiting, I burned the chicken. Oh yeah, and just to top off the day, I broke a dish! The pieces went everywhere."

Jim thought a simple question at this point might be safe enough. "You called the college counselor? What for?" Beth couldn't sit still any longer. She got up and started to walk around the room nervously, tidying up as she spoke. "Oh, I've been worried sick all day thinking about Michael going to college. Sometimes his ADHD seems like it's just getting worse. "Did you know that he forgot to show up for that make-up test in English that I worked so hard to arrange for him?"

Beth paused and sighed again. Jim could feel that they were getting close to the heart of it. Beth finally turned and looked him in the eye as she spoke. "I ran into my friend Annette this morning and I found out that her boy David had to come home from college after less than two months. She's beside herself. She said that they kept hoping that he would somehow outgrow his ADHD problems in college, but here he was home from school almost before he started."

"You know that Annette and I have always joked about how similar Michael and David are. It's not such a funny joke to me right now. I tried not to let this make me crazy, but it kept going round and round in my head, and finally I put in a call to the counselor at school. But, of course, he never called me back and now it's dinner time and I have to eat my burnt chicken and then wait till tomorrow to find out anything."

Jim didn't want to interrupt her now that she was getting to the heart of it, but he was puzzled. "What are you hoping the college counselor can tell you?" "Well, I spent the whole morning on the internet trying to find some advice about sending an ADHD kid to college. There was some talk about finding an "ADHD friendly" college, but I couldn't get straight answers about what "ADHD friendly" really meant, or what to do, or when to do it."

"There were also a lot of other things mentioned that I had never thought about too. Did you know that we may have to have Michael tested again just so he can get extra time on exams in college? Anyway, I spent all that time on the web, and I ended up with more questions than answers. I thought maybe the counselor at school could give me straight answers. But, of course, he never called back."

Jim loved being the answer man at times like this. Which means he also hated it when something like this came up and he didn't feel like he had the answers. He did his best to comfort his wife. He told her that everything would be fine. He didn't tell her about all the worries that he had inside. He didn't mention that he wondered how their boy would even get himself up in the morning at college, much less do all the organizing and planning that his Mom did for him now.

Later that night, they tried the internet again. The next day, they tried again to reach the college counselor at the high school. They did their best. They both wished that there was a simpler way to get answers to all the questions that they had.

****

Does the story you just read sound familiar? Is this a talk that you have had with your spouse? Or maybe you've had a similar conversation with yourself? Or maybe you know you should be thinking about these things but you are just afraid to -- afraid that you will end up like the couple in the story, stuck with a lot of worries and left with more questions than answers.

If so, then this book was written for you.

There are no simple answers when you have a child who has ADHD and it's time to prepare for college. That doesn't mean that there are no answers. As is true with any challenge, information is power. This small book will give you that power. Think of it as a streetwise guide to preparing your ADHD child for the transition to college.

In our work as Clinical Psychologists, we have often worked with ADHD teens and young adults who hope to succeed at college. We have heard the many questions that they and their parents ask about how to prepare for this huge step. We also have learned that these ADHD kids and their families sometimes don't even know what questions to ask.

We have arranged the information in this book in a simple question and answer format. We ask, and then answer, 25 basic questions. Some of these are questions that teens with ADHD and their parent often ask when we meet with them for counseling. Some are questions most ADHD teens and their parents would ask if they only knew a little bit more about ADHD and how it impacts the college experience.

As you might imagine, each of the questions asked here could be answered in a much more detailed way. In fact, there is much more that we would like people to know about this subject. That's why we are planning a series of four books on this topic.

Part one of the series will focus on the transition to college, and part two will focus on thriving at college once you arrive. In part one, you will have this Skinny Book ™, and then a more comprehensive book that covers the same topic in more detail. Similarly, part two will offer a Skinny Book™ and then a more comprehensive book. We believe that this series will be a trustworthy compass to all the teens with ADHD, their families, and all of the professionals who are trying to help them.

We know that you are busy. In the world we live in today, information is plentiful, but wise, concise, well-organized information is hard to find. This Skinny Book™ will provide you with the maximum amount of helpful advice with the minimum amount of time and effort required by you.

So let's get started.

Part I: How to find an ADHD-friendly college

Question 1: What is an ADHD-friendly college?

An ADHD-friendly college is, at the very least, a college where an ADHD student is likely to receive reasonable accommodations and support services that will help the student to be successful at college. In fact, more often than not, when people use a term like "ADHD-friendly", they are probably talking exclusively about the availability of accommodations and services.

In a more general sense, an ADHD-friendly college is simply a college that is a good fit for an ADHD student. ADHD students have particular challenges and needs related to their diagnosis. A college is a good fit if it has characteristics that are likely to be beneficial to the average ADHD student.

For example, ADHD students are often easily distracted. This tendency toward distraction may be reduced when classroom sizes are smaller and when the student is more personally engaged in relationships with classmates and professors. Many ADHD students might therefore do better with smaller colleges that have more intimate classes and more opportunity for personal contact with professors. Other characteristics that might make a college ADHD-friendly will be discussed later in this book.

Although ADHD students can have many things in common, it is also true that each ADHD student is an individual with unique strengths and unique challenges and needs. Therefore, there is no one-size-fits-all definition of ADHD-friendly. Instead, finding an ADHD-friendly college ultimately means finding a college that is a good fit for a particular, unique, ADHD student. This will mean exploring what has worked and what has not worked for the particular individual in the past, and finding a college that is a good fit based on that history.

By the way, the term "ADHD-friendly college" is not an official term with a consensus definition. If you call a college and ask them if they are ADHD-friendly, they may not even know what you are talking about. In later questions we will talk about how to find out if a college is or is not likely to be ADHD-friendly for a particular student.

Question 2: What are "accommodations?"

As you begin to explore the help available at a particular college you may be bewildered by the terminology used. You may wonder about the definition of terms like "accommodations," "adjustments," "modifications," "support services," "resources," and so on. Unfortunately, there are no definitive definitions for some of these terms. In fact, some terms may be used differently or interchangeably at different institutions.

The term "accommodation" is probably the best defined of these terms, and it is generally used in special education to describe an alteration or adjustment that allows individuals with disabilities to participate free from discrimination. In the case of an ADHD student, accommodations are often special conditions, such as extended time on exams, or having a separate room for testing, or being allowed to use a recording device rather than taking notes.

Accommodations are not intended to change basic requirements. They simply allow the student to pursue his or her studies without being unfairly disadvantaged by their disability. The term "modification" is sometimes used, in contrast to the term "accommodations," when there is an actual change in the basic requirements. For example, exempting a student from a college's foreign language requirement would usually be considered a modification because it changes that basic requirement of the college program.

Whatever the vocabulary used at a particular college, there is an important distinction made between help that prevents discrimination and help that tries to insure success. As we will see in the answer to the next question, this is one of the biggest differences between the special education services received from kindergarten to the end of high school and the accommodations and services provided in college.

In short, a college is only required by law to provide help that prevents discrimination. They are not legally required or expected to provide whatever additional services that would be of benefit to assure the success of a student. This means, at minimum, that "accommodations" are appropriate for a college student, but "modifications," which change the nature of the course or school requirements, are not.

Other terms used, such as "services" or "resources" are sometimes attempts to distinguish help that the college is required to provide from help that is not required by law. When help is not required by law, it may not be available, or it may only be available if you pay an extra charge of some kind. For example, "services" is a term sometimes used to refer to things like tutoring or coaching, and at many colleges this is not available directly through the college or, if it is available, you may have to pay extra to receive this kind of help.

Question 3: How do special education services during grade school and high school differ from the kind of help that students receive in college?

There is actually a huge difference in the law that governs special education services from kindergarten through the end of twelfth grade (K-12) and the law that governs the help that students receive in college. Not knowing this simple fact can cause a lot of confusion, false expectations, and problems for students and parents during the transition to college.

During the K-12 years, the law that is most relevant is called the Individuals with Disabilities Education Act, or IDEA. In college, the most relevant law is the Americans with Disabilities Act, or ADA. Actually, it would be more accurate to say that the ADA law always applies, but the IDEA law, which sets a higher standard, does not apply in college. There are important differences between these two laws. The short version is this -- when kids go to college they are not entitled to as much help.

The IDEA law basically states that children should be given a plan and whatever reasonable resources they need in order to succeed in the least restrictive environment. It is the school's responsibility to provide this. This is why a child might have an Individual Educational Plan (or IEP) in grade school or high school. The IEP plan essentially tells how the school is meeting their responsibilities according to the law.

The IDEA law only applies until the end of high school. After that you have only the ADA left, which requires a fair and even playing field. Students must have an equal opportunity to compete, but there is no expectation under the law that the college must go beyond fairness and help the student to succeed.

For example, it can be argued that an ADHD student should be allowed a special testing environment for the same reason that a person in a wheel chair should have wheel chair accessible classrooms. Without such adjustments to create equal opportunity, it could be said that the individuals with ADHD would be subject to discrimination due to his or her disability.

However, the school does not need to provide a tutor. Even if a tutor would really, really help the student to succeed, it is just not the requirement of the college, under the law, to provide something like that. In contrast, the same child in high school might have had help from special education teachers who provided, within reason, whatever the child needed.

In practice, it is sometimes not clear what kind of help serves to level the playing field and what goes beyond and aims at maximizing potential. Some might argue that a tutor for an ADHD student does level the playing field in much the same way that a ramp levels the playing field for a physically disabled student, but this does not appear to be the interpretation under the law at present.

The change from IDEA to ADA has a couple of other important implications. First, K-12 schools actually get government funding to implement the requirements of IDEA. Colleges, in contrast, do not get any money from the government to implement ADA. They are simply required to obey the ADA laws if they want to get any other funding from the government, which will be the case for almost all colleges. As we will see in the next question, this means that colleges will decide for themselves what they want to provide as part of standard tuition, and what extra services they feel they need to provide in order to be in compliance with the law.

A second important implication of the change from IDEA to ADA is that it becomes the responsibility of the student to seek out the help that is available. This means first that the burden of proof is on the student to provide evidence of a disability. The college does not have to test the student. Then, if and when the college agrees that the student has a disability, it is the student's job to find out what help is available and to utilize it.

Question 4: If the law determines what kind of help is given, why are there differences from one college to another?

Some colleges may do the absolute minimum that they need to do in order to comply with the law. Even when a college chooses to do the minimum, there is no absolute formula that determines that minimum. Therefore, even schools that have decided to do the absolute minimum may differ in what they believe the minimum is: some may responsibly do the minimum while others might try to interpret the law in the stingiest way possible, with their only concern being that they might be challenged under the law.

For example, one school may be more strict than another about what proof of disability a student must submit in order to be granted accommodations. Alternatively, one school might be more conservative than others in the types of accommodations that they allow.

Then there are colleges that offer more than the legal minimum. These schools may vary greatly in how far they choose to exceed the minimum requirements in terms of offering free accommodations and services. Then there are also colleges that offer some services for a fee, and of course, there will be differences in what they offer and how much they charge.

In the end, you have a spectrum of possible services ranging from the minimum required by law at one extreme, all the way to very comprehensive well-designed programs that are offered for ADHD college students.

Question 5: Are there basic categories that colleges fall into with regard to the kind of help that they offer?

There are no official categories. However, some professionals have tried, in books or websites for example, to give a general overview of what kind of accommodations and services are offered. These professionals sometimes talk about three categories or levels of accommodations and services offered. The categories offered by different professionals may not line up exactly, but there are broad similarities.

At one extreme, you have colleges that are offering the minimum help, or close to the minimum help, that is required by law. At the other extreme, you have colleges that make a reasonable attempt to offer a variety of services that might benefit a student with a disability. Then you have colleges in-between these two extremes, offering something beyond the minimum required by law, but not attempting to offer the broad variety of services that might be of benefit to an ADHD student.

When professionals organize colleges into levels or categories, they are basically talking about the three groups of colleges that we have been discussing -- the colleges offering the minimum in order to level the playing field, the colleges offering the maximum in order to promote success, and the colleges that fall between these two extremes.

These different categories may be given different names by different professionals. We will refer to these three categories using the terms "Basic services," "Intermediate services" and "Complete services". We will summarize some of the differences between types of help offered at different colleges using these three terms.

As you might imagine, the middle category, which we refer to as "intermediate services" is the most difficult to characterize accurately. This category, by definition, spans a range from one extreme of services to the other. However, in practice, most colleges tend to be nearer to the minimal services end of the spectrum. Therefore, when we discuss "intermediate services" below, we will focus on what is typical. The typical intermediate services college provides more than basic services, but not a lot more.

These descriptions are intended as general guidelines, not rules written in stone. A given school will not necessarily fit one category in all ways. Categories can help to provide an overview of what is offered so as to make it easier to navigate that complex world of college choices out there. Remember, these are not official categories. If you ask a school what category they are in, they probably won't know what you are talking about.

Table 1: Categories of Services Provided by Colleges

Category	Basic	Intermediate	Complete
Goal of Disability Support Services	To provide minimum services required by law.	To provide more than the minimum services required by law.	To provide most or all service that might benefit students, going well beyond what is required by law.
Office for Disability Support Services	Typically not a separate office. Disability services are probably provided by an individual who has other job responsibilities.	There may be a dedicated office of disability support services and one or more professionals dedicated to serving disable students.	There is a dedicated office and staff members have special training and experience related to working with students needing services.
Funds available	Typically little or no money is provided by the college for disability services.	Minimal or moderate funds are provided by the college.	Substantial funds are provided by the college and/or acquired through fees.
Formal Policies and Procedures for Providing Services	Typically no formal policies or procedures are established.	There are some minimal formal policies and procedures in place.	More substantial formal policies and procedures are in place.

Category	Basic	Intermediate	Complete
Responsibility to Find and Access Information and Services	It is entirely the student's responsibility, and the system may be difficult to navigate.	Although the responsibility is still primarily on the student to seek out services, trained professionals will facilitate students once they do seek services.	There is often a "wrap-around" approach - meaning that the staff takes more responsibility for reaching out to the student and maintaining contact and helping students to find and utilize the available services.

You might think, given the summaries above, that a college with complete services is better than one with intermediate services, which is better than one with basic services. That is not necessarily true. The rule is that more services are generally better, but there are at least two important exceptions to that rule.

The first exception is that sometimes comprehensive services might be overkill for a particular student. If the student only needs a little extra help, then the hand-holding of a truly comprehensive program might seem oppressive to the student. The case management approach of a college that offers more complete services might smother a student that really only needs a particular accommodation during exams.

The second exception has to do with cost. It may be that the complete program would be better for a particular student in a perfect world. But that is kind of like saying that living in a mansion is better than living in a minimal apartment. Most people living in minimal apartments would say, "yeah, I know that, but I can't afford to live in a mansion." Making choices about what services a particular student needs will, similarly, need to take the financial realities into consideration.

Question 6: How do I find out which schools might have good programs for ADHD students?

There are two excellent resources that can be invaluable as you begin your search:

* K & W Guide to Colleges for Students with Learning Disabilities or Attention Deficit Hyperactivity Disorder. (10th Edition.) By Princeton Review, by authors Marybeth Kravets M.A. and Imy F. Wax M.S.

* Peterson's Colleges for Students with Learning Disabilities or ADD. (8th Edition.)
(also see www.petersons.com for a search engine that will generate a list of schools based on specific criteria.)

As of the writing of this book, the most recent version of the K & W book is published in 2010, while the latest version of the Peterson's guide is from 2007. We recommend the K & W book because it is currently more up to date, but both books are excellent.

Question 7: Are there scholarships available to ADHD students?

Here is an excellent article that provides a summary of scholarships available for students with ADHD:

http://add.about.com/od/adhdresources/a/Scholarships.htm

Question 8: If I find an "ADHD-friendly" college, will my child be okay?

Unfortunately, there is no college that can guarantee any student's success. This is true with or without ADHD. College students with ADHD face a number of challenges related to their diagnosis. In addition to academic problems, students with ADHD often face many other challenges, including emotional issues, social issues, and difficulties in other areas. No college can provide a perfect answer to these many challenges.

There are other things, besides picking a good college, that can be done to help an ADHD teen make a good transition to college. We will discuss some of the things that might be done in the next question. However, we must acknowledge from the start that it will never be possible to guarantee success for all ADHD college students, even though there are many things that can be done to dramatically increase the probability of success for the average ADHD college student. There are several reasons that this is true.

First, ADHD can have a powerful impact on the college experience. Many underestimate this impact, thinking that ADHD simply impairs academic performance in some relatively minor way. In reality, the impact of ADHD is considerable and ADHD creates both academic and non-academic difficulties.

There are, frankly, important differences in terms of the degree of challenge faced by different teens with ADHD. For some, it could be unrealistic to expect that they will succeed at college even if they are trying hard and they are given the advantage of every possible form of help. We believe that this is rarely the case, but the possibility cannot be dismissed. Even with teens that have no disability, college is not the right choice for all.

The degree to which the teen with ADHD acknowledges the problems and works diligently to address them will also be a factor. We would never simply blame ADHD teens for their problems, any more than we would blame a visually impaired individual for needing glasses. However, as almost anyone with a disability will tell you, there is always a question of how hard the disabled person works to recognize and address a disability.

We hope, in other books in this series, to provide skills and strategies that help prepare the college bound ADHD student from the inside out, so as to maximize the probability of college success. Ultimately, the only way to keep a child safe near water is to teach them to swim. Similarly, an essential part of helping an ADHD student to succeed is to teach him skills and strategies that will allow him to better meet the unique challenges he will face.

Question 9: Other than accommodations and services available, what other factors might make a college ADHD-friendly?

As mentioned earlier, each ADHD individual is unique, so ultimately this question must be answered after taking the unique aspects of the individual student into account. However, there are some general principles that might be helpful to the average ADHD student and it is in that spirit that we offer the following suggestions.

1. Consider smaller more intimate colleges.

As mentioned earlier, ADHD college students will have difficulties with distraction. Colleges that have smaller class size and more chance to interact directly with professors and instructors may minimize the tendency to be distracted. Sitting in a giant auditorium, perhaps with nobody that you know personally, listening to a professor that you may never speak to personally, may be quite the norm in large universities. However, this is not the ideal environment for someone who is easily distracted.

Our experience is that ADHD individuals do better academically when the material to be learned is presented in a way that feels more personally relevant. This is probably true for everyone to a degree, but it is often dramatically true for individuals with ADHD. Having this feeling that the material is personally relevant is more likely when the student has a realer connection to the teacher and the others in the class.

Some have suggested that ADHD students might actually do better at bigger colleges because they are likely to be bored by the smaller college environment. The argument here seems to be that the student must be happy with the college experience in general or feelings of boredom or irritability with tend to increase symptoms like distractibility and impulsivity.

Our experience suggests that this would not be the best overall choice for most ADHD students. However, it may be true for some, and is probably a good example of how the individual characteristics of the student must be considered in deciding what makes a school truly ADHD - friendly.

2. Explore the curriculum and look for requirements that might be problematic.

Remember, one of the big differences between high school and college with regard to the help students with ADHD get is that colleges are less likely to soften the actual school requirements. The college must allow the ADHD student to compete fairly, but they do not have to modify the basic requirements.

For example, ADHD students sometimes have difficulty with a particular subject, such as math or foreign language. In high school, it may have been possible to change the curriculum in some way or even exempt the student from a course that would otherwise be expected.

This will usually not be an option in a college environment. Therefore, it makes sense to look ahead and see what the school requires. For example, if the ADHD student has a history of great difficulty with foreign language, it makes sense to find a school that either does not have a foreign language requirement or is one of the rare colleges that allows ADHD students some flexibility in meeting the requirement. Alternatively, if other factors make a school with such a requirement worth considering, you might want to be ready to utilize tutoring to support the student proactively rather than waiting for a problem to develop.

Similarly, try to come up with an inventory of what might be vulnerabilities for the student in question, and then explore the college curriculum to see if those vulnerabilities are particularly problematic at this college. Some things to consider might be foreign language, math, and the need to write papers.

It would also make sense to see what the policy is regarding attendance. Some schools may make class attendance mandatory with serious consequences if you have more than one or two absences. This can be a formula for disaster for some ADHD students.

There is, or course, a trade off with regard to mandatory attendance. Some students might be less likely to go to class knowing that attendance is not mandatory. This could quickly turn into a problem for an impulsive ADHD student. At the same time, in our opinion, a very rigid policy regarding attendance is more likely to be a curse than a blessing for an ADHD student.

3. <u>Evaluate the housing options available</u>.

Housing is an important factor in the college experience of any young person, but this is dramatically truer for the ADHD student. There are a number of factors to consider here. Is it better to have a single room or better to have a roommate? If the college is close to home, (or close to a relative's home,) is it better to live at home or on campus? Is it better to live on campus in a dorm or find a place to rent near school? What about fraternities and sororities?

How do you minimize the possible negative aspects of living situations, such as drugs and alcohol, or just the distraction of constant access to social interaction? What living arrangement is the best fit given the student's feelings about staying up late or having a clean living space?

There are no easy answers to questions like those noted above, but we will try to briefly spell out some of the pros and cons of different choices here, and we will deal with this topic in a little more detail in the companion book in the series. Our main point here, in this book, is that you should do an inventory of costs and benefits of housing options, taking ADHD issues into account.

At many colleges, freshmen will be required to live in the dorms and have at least one roommate. Living with a roommate is a challenge for anyone, but when you have ADHD there are some additional things to consider.

ADHD students may sometimes have social difficulties. From poor social skills, to anger issues, to being messy, to forgetting for the umpteenth time that your roommate asked you not to do that drumming thing with your pencil while you're studying -- there are many reasons that ADHD college students might clash with roommates.

In addition, ADHD students often do, even more than college students in general, have difficulty staying with a "regular" schedule. If the student in question is an ADHD night owl, living with a roommate may be even more of an issue.

Last, but not least, a roommate is a distraction, and ADHD students already have enough trouble with distractions. It may be very difficult to study with a roommate nearby listening to music or talking on the phone or even entertaining a friend. It is even more distracting if they keep telling you that you should join them and put off your studying for later.

The other side of this coin is that students who live in single rooms or off campus in apartments can become socially isolated. The dorm life is an important part of how college kids make friends. Realistically, academic challenges are not the only reason that college students have trouble making it through freshman year. If the student is miserable socially, the student will not want to stay, and their grades will likely plummet over time in any event.

Sometimes a roommate can also be a good example, and even,

you might say, an anti-distraction. Seeing your roommate study every night at a certain time might help you to get down to work yourself.

Although there is no perfect answer, most ADHD students would, in our opinion, benefit from a single room that is not too removed from other students, such as a single room in a dorm, or an apartment shared with one or more others but with private rooms.

For students that really need a lot of support, it may be best to find a commuter college that is near to home, or near to the home of a relative or friend. This extra support might be useful throughout the college years, or it may be needed only in order to get through a transition period, such as the first year.

If you feel that a single room would be the best option, but that is difficult or impossible to find, you will need to find ways of minimizing the possible problems associated with roommates. We will address this topic in more detail in the companion book.

4. <u>Try to find out if the college has a reputation as a party school</u>.

ADHD students are, on average, more at risk for substance abuse issues and impulsive behavior regarding sexuality. Although drugs and alcohol are available at most colleges, there are some colleges with a reputation for being on the wild side. These schools add even more temptation and distraction to the ADHD student's already very full dance card. It is probably not a good idea to include these schools on your short list of options.

5. <u>Explore options at the school for simplifying day-to-day challenges.</u>

We're talking here about meal plans rather than cooking on your own; having laundry services nearby rather than farther away; having a medical center nearby; being near a library or quiet place to study; having an easy place to refill medications; and so on.

Anton Chekhov said, "Any idiot can face a crisis, it's the day to day living that wears you out." This may be true for all of us, but it is even truer when you have ADHD. Anything you can do to simplify the life of an ADHD college student improves the likelihood of a positive college experience.

Question 10: What else (besides college choice) will help an ADHD teen make a good transition to college?

There are many things that might help an ADHD teen make a better transition to college. Ideally, high school students could be working gradually from early in the high school years to develop skills that will help with this transition. In this skinny book we will assume that most or all readers are already nearing the end of high school and are currently facing the college application and admissions process. This means that you have a year or so left to make preparations for the transition.

We will touch on several things that can be done now, whether you are a college bound student with ADHD, or the parent of such a student, or a professional working with such a student. We will address the details of these things that you can do in later questions (e.g.; see questions 22, 23 and 24 below) and in our companion book as well. For now, our goal is simply to provide an overview.

> 1. A foundation of a good transition is a good understanding of what ADHD is and how it might impact the college experience. This includes having an understanding of how symptoms and challenges of ADHD might change as people move from childhood into adulthood. It is important that college bound students who have ADHD have a realistic understanding of their disorder and a motivation to do what they can to prepare for success in college.

> 2. In addition, it is important that parents of college bound ADHD students also have a good understanding of what

ADHD is and how it might affect the college experience. Parents and their college bound children should also work to enhance communication and to clarify how parents and the student should interact during the college years. In particular, there should, ideally, be some consensus regarding what role parents will play during this transition.

An attempt should be made to clear the air regarding disagreements about the disorder, the parent's role in helping, power struggles that may have become entrenched, and so on.

3. If there are services that might be of benefit during college that are not offered by the college that has been chosen, some attempt could be made to find and provide those services independently. For example, a student might be connected to a counselor or an ADHD life coach, or someone teaching study skills, or a tutor. Costs of such services could be explored and included to some degree in budgeting for college.

In this way, a college that offers basic services or intermediate services could, in effect, be upgraded by creatively adding services provided privately. This could be particularly useful in helping during a set transition period, such as the first two months, or the first semester, to increase the possibility of getting off to a good start. For many, this will be more financially realistic than a fully supportive (but expensive) program.

4. If possible, the student might meet with a counselor or coach for a period during the end of high school in order to get professional help in identifying strengths and challenges and devising a plan for picking the best school and addressing possible transition challenges. If the student already is receiving counseling services, the counselor or coach could be asked to work on these goals. The student could also work on stress and emotion management skills during this period.

5. As mentioned earlier, finding an ADHD-friendly college can mean more than just finding out what services are provided by the college. A more comprehensive approach attempts to find a good match with regard to several variables, including how near or far from home the school is, what kind of living arrangements are possible, are there siblings or other family members or friends nearby that can provide support, and so on.

6. Even if there is not a lot of time left before the student will leave for college, some steps could be taken to teach and practice life skills before the student is alone and overwhelmed by many other challenges. Have the student practice doing his or her own laundry. Have them handle money in some way that approximates the skills they will need at school. Have them be more responsible for getting themselves up in the morning, or other responsibilities that parents may regularly provide assistance at present. In short, wean the young person from their dependence on parents or others before they are suddenly all on their own.

7. Explore medication options. If the student is not on medications, make sure you have accurate information before assuming that avoiding medication is the best option. If the student is already on medication, see if there might be a better way of taking medication at college. It may make sense to take the medication later in the day, or use a newer alternative method such as a patch. In college, one could anticipate that the needs for attentiveness and focus during studying will extend much longer into the evening hours. This may require a change in medication strategy.

8. Explore alternatives that might support better symptom management. For example, some believe that poor nutrition and lack of exercise can make symptoms worse. This includes caution about use of nicotine, caffeine,

sugar, and over-the-counter drugs. Similarly, look at ways to encourage proper sleep. Consider vitamins and other supplements that might help.

9. If parents and student are both in agreement, it may be possible for parents to help, at least to some degree, even from a distance. For example, parents might text at a particular time every day to remind the student to take medication. A schedule, detailing classes and study periods, might be prepared as soon as classes are chosen. Weekend phone calls or emails might be utilized to talk about and monitor how longer term projects can be organized and broken down into steps.

Parents should not hover or intervene any more than necessary. As mentioned earlier, there should be some consensus between parents and student regarding what would be help and what would be a nuisance. There should also be a plan to wean the student of such support as much as possible and as soon as possible as the college years progress.

At the same time, there should be a realistic acknowledgement that many college bound students with ADHD will need some extra support. It should also be noted that parents have some right to be involved until the student demonstrates an ability to do these things independently given that the parents will be affected both financially and in other ways if the student overestimates their ability to act independently.

Question 11: Is a school that had good services for learning disabilities also a good school for an ADHD child?

Although the answer is probably yes, there is no guarantee, so it is a good idea to explicitly check and evaluate how ADHD friendly a given college is. Many individuals with ADHD will also have Learning Disabilities (LD), but ADHD is definitely not the same thing as LD.

As a general rule, young people with LD will be better at accessing and utilizing resources that are provided by the college. These individuals may have problems with processing certain kinds of materials, but they do not necessarily have the kinds of difficulties that ADHD students have with executive functioning.

For example, if you have a young person who has difficulty writing papers due to learning disabilities, a writing lab provided by the college where students are given help with papers may be very useful. On the other hand, the young person with ADHD is likely to have significant executive functioning problems. If they are told about the writing lab, they may forget to go, or fail to use the tools provided at the lab, or fail to hand their paper in even if they complete it.

If people at the college disability office have specialized training only in Learning Disabilities and not ADHD, they may not always know how to help an ADHD student. They may, in fact, fall into the same trap that other adults in the young ADHD person's life have -- of failing to recognize ADHD symptoms and instead thinking that the person has a flawed character.

So, you might ask, why do we start our answer by saying "the answer is probably yes?" Because, practically speaking, schools that invest heavily in providing excellent programs for students with LD will likely have staff with some knowledge of ADHD. In fact, students with LD will so often also have ADHD, that it would be kind of negligent to train someone in LD without also training them to know at least something about ADHD.

Simply know that the resources that will help an LD student may not be as much help for an ADHD student. It is always a good idea to ask whether the staff at Disability Services has special training or expertise regarding ADHD. The more severe the symptoms of ADHD of a given student, the more important this becomes. A student with mild ADHD may be able to utilize that writing lab we mentioned earlier, but a student with severe symptoms may need much more support.

Part II: When, where and how to contact colleges regarding ADHD

Question 12: Whom do I contact at the college to talk about accommodations and services provided for students with ADHD?

At many colleges, there will be a dedicated office of Disability Support Services. This is usually the place to contact. Sometimes the office that handles disability support services has a different name, such as "Office of Student Disability Services," or just "Disability Services," or some other similar name.

As a general rule, call and ask first for the Office of Disability Services. If they don't have one, ask who handles accommodations for students with ADHD. You may be given an office with a similar sounding name, though some schools will not have a dedicated office for handling students with disabilities at all. If this is the case, you will be put in contact with a person who handles disability services, but there will be no dedicated office.

Question 13: When should I first make contact with the college disability office?

Ideally, your college search should incorporate a strategy for finding an ADHD-friendly school from the very beginning. This means determining what level of services you believe you will likely need and finding colleges that are able to provide those services.

We suggest therefore that students contact the Offices of Disability Services during their junior year when they are deciding to which colleges they will apply. We would suggest using guide books and other resource to first make an initial list of potential colleges that includes twice as many colleges as you would actually like to apply to. Then contact their Offices of Disability Services and ask some questions to thin out your list. This will leave you with a final list of schools to which you will actually apply. (We will talk about what questions to ask later in this book.)

Unfortunately, many students simply apply to schools initially based on academic qualities and personal preferences and wait until they are admitted before exploring ADHD resources. This is a terrible strategy. What good is an otherwise excellent school if it does not provide the support that will allow an ADHD student to succeed?

Question 14: How much do the professionals at the disability office know about ADHD?

That will depend on the school. Schools will vary dramatically in this regard. Some will have professionals handling disability services without any specialized training. At other schools, professionals will have some training, but they may still not have much knowledge of ADHD. For example, sometimes the professional in charge will know a lot about Learning Disabilities, but will have little or no expertise regarding ADHD.

Because of this variability in training, we encourage students and those assisting them to inquire directly about the ADHD training/expertise of the professionals handling disability services. Specific questions to ask will be considered below.

Question 15: Can I use the fact that my child has and IEP in high school to prove that he or she needs accommodations in college?

Usually the answer will be no. Although you probably can use the

IEP as part of the evidence that you provide, this evidence will usually not be enough. In another answer below we will outline the evidence that often is required. (See question # 17.)

Question 16: Can I have a Psychiatrist or other professional working with my child write a letter in order to prove that he or she needs accommodations in college?

Sometimes, but very likely the answer will be no. Colleges will have specific requirements as to what you need to do in order to be granted disability status based on ADHD. We will discuss common requirements in some detail in a question below, but a letter from a professional will often not be enough. In fact, as more and more students with ADHD are applying for accommodations at colleges, it is likely that the requirements for demonstrating a need will get more and more rigorous.

Question 17: What is needed in order for a college student to be granted disability status based on ADHD so as to be allowed access to the modifications and services provided by the college?

We will outline the most common requirements, but it should be noted that colleges may differ in terms of their requirements and their timetable for submitting required documents. It is necessary to check in with the Office of Disability Services at each school to determine their requirements.

In general, here is what you will need to provide in order to be eligible for accommodations and services at a college.

1. <u>Documentation has to be current.</u> You will need to contact the school regarding what they consider current, and whether they make exceptions if you have an evaluation

that just misses their cutoff point. The main point here is that a childhood evaluation probably will not be sufficient.

Colleges have the right to insist that an evaluation demonstrate that the student currently is disabled in a way and to a degree that justifies the accommodations and services requested. This means it must be age appropriate and show evidence of the current level of functioning.

2. <u>An evaluation must be provided by a qualified professional.</u> This generally means a licensed physician or mental health professional, but again, you need to check with the college to see what they consider acceptable. There is some debate in the field regarding who is and is not qualified to provide an assessment of ADHD.

   The professional should have direct experience with the student. This means, for example, that you probably cannot have someone simply write a report based upon existing documents or previous test results. Again, each college may have their own requirements regarding the degree of direct experience the professional must have had with the student in order to provide the examination, so check with them.

3. <u>A diagnosis should be included.</u> This means that specific symptoms that lead to a diagnosis (based on the current version of the Diagnostic and Statistical Manual, or DSM) must be included. More to the point, you may be denied if, instead of a diagnosis, there are "indications of ADHD," or "a pattern suggesting ADHD," or other vague references in place of a definitive diagnosis.

4. <u>Relevant test data should be included.</u> Often colleges will want to verify for themselves, based on the actual test data, that the diagnosis and recommendations are valid. A

professional often cannot simply provide a letter stating that "testing was done", and certain conclusions were reached.

This means that, for some schools, your Pediatrician or Pediatric Psychiatrist may not be able to provide the information that you need. Medical professionals do routinely diagnose ADHD, but they usually do so based on a diagnostic interview. They may not supplement that diagnostic interview with formal test data.

5. <u>Recommendations regarding specific accommodations and services being requested should be provided.</u> Again, the fact that a student received certain accommodations in high school is simply not enough to grant similar accommodations in college. The reasons for each accommodation, and the evidence supporting that request, may be required before anything is granted.

Each school has its own rules with regard to what is required. You should certainly inquire as to what documentation is needed, and by whom, and by what date, with each college to which you are applying. It makes little sense to pick a school based on the wonderful disability services they provide if it is unlikely that they will, in the end, provide those services in your individual case.

What all of this means is you may need to have a mental health professional provide a current evaluation with the express purpose of providing appropriate evidence to colleges. Unfortunately, this could mean spending hundreds of dollars to prove something that you feel you already know.

However, this may be a valuable investment if such accommodations or access to special services leads to the success of your child. In addition, a current assessment may show changes that have developed since the last testing and this may allow for more fine-tuned interventions during the college years.

Question 18: If my child says something about their ADHD during the application process, could that be used as a basis for not accepting them into the college?

Legally, the college is not allowed to discriminate. Nonetheless, the real answer is probably that there is no way to know for sure. Many people, including professionals working in college admissions, may have misunderstandings and biases about ADHD. This could conceivably influence a decision, even if the professional is not consciously intending to discriminate.

Although there is no way to know for sure, we believe that it would be a rarity in this day and age for college admissions professionals to have such a negative view of ADHD and even rarer that they would allow it to influence their decision given that they are not legally allowed to discriminate. Furthermore, as we will discuss in upcoming questions, there can be good reasons to talk about a history of ADHD on an application.

Question 19: If my child seeks help for ADHD during college, will that information be available in the future to employers?

That information will be kept confidential. The Americans with Disabilities Law requires that such information be kept confidential.

Question 20: What, if anything, should my child say about their disability during the application process?

Sometimes talking about ADHD in the application process could provide an advantage. The clearest example of this is when there is a history of academic problems and then a turnaround occurs when the child is diagnosed and begins to receive medication and/or counseling. If the admissions committee does not know about the ADHD, they will only see the problems in the academic record. If they hear about the ADHD they have the story of a young person who faced a challenge and then addressed the challenge successfully.

Admissions committees are not allowed to soften admission criteria for a person with a disability. However, they may, for example, view a poor freshman year more favorably if it is seen as due to a disability that is now being addressed. In such a case, a failure to disclose the full history may leave the admissions committee with the view that the child had some failure in terms of discipline or motivation or some other character flaw.

Similarly, if there is any gap or deficiency in the student's record, you have to ask yourself if the correct explanation is better than the explanation an admissions committee might come up with in a vacuum. Ultimately the question is, "Will the overall story of the person be enhanced if the challenges of ADHD are acknowledged and addressed in the application?"

However, it should be noted that there is a balancing act here too. Remember that colleges are not allowed to discriminate due to any disability, but neither are they required to modify basic requirements for admissions. For example, imagine that you have a student who was allowed to not take a foreign language in high school, because their ADHD made that course particularly difficult.

On the one hand, the college may be more understanding about the lack of foreign language on the high school transcript if they know that it is related to a history of ADHD. On the other hand, if the college does have its own foreign language requirement that cannot be modified, they will have a right to note this as a weakness.

Question 21: What questions should I ask the college to find out if the school is ADHD-friendly?

The list of questions offered below is intended to help you gather information. These questions are not intended to be litmus tests that must be answered positively in order to consider the school.

However, the more evidence that the needs of ADHD students have been carefully considered the better.

Contact the Office of Disability Support Services, (or the professional who handles accommodations for students with ADHD if there is no office dedicated to disability services,) and ask the following questions, as summarized in Table 2.

Table 2. Questions to Ask at the College

#	Question to Ask	Yes	No	N/A	Comments or Notes
1	Do the staff members at the disability services office have any special training or expertise that qualifies them to work with ADHD students?				
2	Is there an established process to qualify for accommodations?				
3	Is there a defined timeframe to apply for accommodations?				
	When do we need to apply for such accommodations?				
	Who needs to provide an evaluation, including qualifications of evaluator?				
	What elements need to be included in the evaluation?				

4	Is there a defined time limit to what is considered to be a current evaluation?			
	What is considered a current evaluation (within how many months?)			
5	Does the school offer special accommodations for students with ADHD?			
	Extended time for exams?			
	Note takers?			
	Special environments for testing?			
	Use of recording devices?			
	Laptops or Tablets?			
	Alternative formats for exams?			
	Other accommodations?			
6	Are there any special services or resources available to ADHD students?			
	Specialized tutors?			
	Writing labs?			
	Math labs?			
	ADHD support groups?			
	ADHD coaching?			

	Other means of helping with time-management, organizational or study skills?			
	Other means of helping with emotional problems?			
7	Can an ADHD student get priority housing in receiving a single room?			
8	Is there a housekeeping service available for room cleaning?			
	What is the charge for this service?			
9	Is there a laundry service available?			
	What is the charge for this service?			
10	Can an ADHD student get early or priority registration for classes?			
11	If a student has difficulty in a particular academic area (such as math or foreign language), is there any flexibility with regard to meeting degree requirements?			

12	If there is flexibility with academic requirements, what procedure must be followed before one is allowed to be exempted or make a substitution? For example, does the student have to fail a course before they can apply for substitution?			
13	Are faculty educated regarding ADHD accommodations and does the Office of Disability Services help the student communicate with faculty?			
14	Will the Office of Disability Services negotiate disputes if any arise?			
15	Are there any ADHD students that work with the Office of Disability Services that can be contacted to discuss their experiences at the school?			
16	Are the services for Learning Disabled students and the services for ADHD students identical?			
	If there are distinct services designed for ADHD students, what are they?			

17	How long has the Office of Disability Services been in existence?	
18	How many staff members are there?	
19	How long have the various staff members been working at the office?	
	Director	
	Head Psychologist	
	Head Social Worker	
20	Is there a staff member that is dedicated to ADHD students?	
	What are this professional's credentials (MD, PsyD, PhD, LCSW, etc.)?	

Part III: Understanding ADHD and its impact on the college experience

Question 22: Don't people outgrow ADHD as they move into adulthood?

Most people do not outgrow ADHD. The estimates for how many children outgrow ADHD vary, but a common estimate is that at least two thirds of children continue to have significant symptoms after high school.

Although most do not outgrow ADHD, the symptoms may change for many as they move into adulthood. For some, the symptoms of hyperactivity tend to lessen as they grow up. Since many people incorrectly believe that hyperactivity is the main or only symptom of ADHD, it is not surprising that people also believe that it is common to outgrow ADHD.

Unfortunately, the symptoms of impulsivity and inattention generally continue into adulthood, and symptoms of hyperactivity sometimes do. You might say that ADHD in adulthood sometimes goes underground. It may be less visible except to those who are trained in symptom identification.

Sadly, the symptoms of adult ADHD, even more than the childhood symptoms, may leave others with a negative view of the ADHD individual. People usually won't see the symptoms as symptoms. They may think that they are seeing laziness, or someone who doesn't care, or selfishness. In other words, they may see the symptoms of ADHD as evidence that the individual is not a good person.

In fact, it may be that ADHD causes more serious problems in adulthood than it does during childhood. This is not due to the disorder getting worse. Rather, it is because the normal transition to adulthood, in which help from others decreases and individual responsibilities increase, is simply more difficult for those with ADHD.

During childhood and adolescence, young people have the support of parents and extended family members as well as teachers, clergy, coaches and others. For a child with ADHD this is dramatically truer, and it often takes a village to get them through the school years successfully and into young adulthood.

As the ADHD child moves into the years after high school, they will, like other young people, begin to do more and more for themselves. Unlike most other young people, they may find this transition overwhelming. The ongoing symptoms of ADHD can wreak havoc as young people try to take on more and more adult responsibility.

In many ways, ADHD is related to problems with what are sometimes called "executive functions." Think about what an executive does in a corporation. The executive does all of the organizing and planning. The executive sees the big picture. The executive sets the goals and creates the steps to achieve those goals. Executive functioning means, in a broad sense, being in charge of your life.

When you have difficulty with executive functioning, as people with ADHD do, sometimes it can feel like nobody is in charge. Nobody is doing all of that planning and organizing. Nobody is visualizing the future and seeing the costs and benefits of taking different paths. Nobody is setting goals. Nobody is in charge of saying, "hey, we have to do something right now that is not very fun so that we can have a good future later on." Sometimes it feels like being in a car going really fast but with nobody in the driver's seat.

As a result, young adults with ADHD are at risk in a number of areas. They are less likely to finish high school, less likely to go to college, and probably more likely to have difficulty at college if they do go. They also are more likely to have problems with money, more likely to be involved with drugs, more likely to get pregnant or get someone pregnant, and more likely to have problems with the law.

If you look at all the many ways that adults with ADHD seem to be impacted by their symptoms, it appears that adult ADHD is actually a pretty serious disorder. It may create more challenges than other major psychiatric problems such as anxiety disorders and depressive (mood) disorders.

So no, kids do not outgrow ADHD. This is a real and challenging disorder that needs to be taken seriously. If anything, it should perhaps be taken more seriously during the young adult years.

The good news, and the bad news, is that many of the problems associated with ADHD in adulthood may be due to people not knowing enough about it and not treating it as seriously as they should. That is bad news because a lot of people are suffering. It is good news because a given individual can likely change their future dramatically for the better by getting good information and taking effective action based on that information.

Question 23: I've heard that ADHD is not even a real disorder -- that it is just a way for drug companies and others to make money by convincing people that they have a "disorder" and then selling them a medication. Is this true?

ADHD is unquestionably a real disorder. There is an overwhelming consensus among professionals that the disorder is real, and that it can be quite challenging. There are even very real differences that show up in the brain when using brain imaging methods. It is clear that ADHD is not simply due to laziness, or bad parenting. It is not simply a sign of a society that tries to make people conform if they don't fit some mold. In fact, the evidence that ADHD is a real disorder is so overwhelming, it is amazing that these myths gain any traction at all.

It is natural that people might want to believe that they do not have a real disorder, People would, of course, prefer to believe that they do not need to learn about ADHD and do all the work of learning to manage it effectively. Similarly, it is also natural for parents and other relatives to want to believe that ADHD is not real. Myths about ADHD gain traction, in part, because people want to believe in them so badly.

ADHD is real and it can cause serious difficulties if it is not managed effectively. The myths that exist denying the validity of ADHD are not just wrong, they can be dangerous. They can be dangerous because they feed into people's desire to deny their disorder, and this prevents people from taking the steps that they could take to create a better and more fulfilling life with ADHD.

Question 24: Doesn't focusing too much on ADHD hurt a young adult's confidence and self-esteem?

More often, the opposite is true. Nothing is more devastating to a young adult's self-esteem than believing that the symptoms of ADHD are really just character flaws. As mentioned earlier, ADHD symptoms can make an individual seem to be lazy or selfish or lacking in some other aspect of character.

When a person is physically disabled, people usually see the disability and do not blame them for the ways that the disability limits them. Nobody in a wheelchair is seen as lazy. A blind person is not seen as uncaring if they bump into you. But with ADHD, people often do not recognize or understand the disorder. Children and adults with ADHD are often seen in a negative light because of this.

Over time, individuals with ADHD may come to see themselves in a negative way because of the way they experience the world. It may seem like people are always mad at them or disappointed with them. It's hard not to see yourself in a negative light when the world keeps reacting to you in a negative way.

One of the best books out there for individuals with ADHD, written by Kate Kelly and Peggy Ramundo, is titled "You mean I'm not lazy, stupid or crazy?" We've lost track of the number of young people we've worked with who have discovered this book and expressed relief and dramatically increased self-esteem after reading it.

The title of the book by Kelly and Ramundo brilliantly captures the feeling many have growing up with ADHD. The feeling is that there must be something terribly wrong with me and it must be my fault. When children and adults with whom we have worked find out that they have ADHD, and understand the ways it can make you look or feel "lazy, stupid or crazy," they feel a tremendous sense of relief. One young man we worked with likened it to having DNA evidence proving a murderer innocent after years of being in prison.

It is true that some individuals with ADHD may feel uncomfortable with the diagnosis. They would rather not have any of the symptoms of ADHD. They would rather not have to do the work of learning about ADHD and finding ways of managing it. But they don't have the luxury of just not having ADHD. Not talking about it does not make it go away.

Really, young people with ADHD have two choices. The first choice is to feel bad about themselves because they have the problems that ADHD causes but they don't realize how ADHD is impacting them and/or they don't know what to do about it. The second choice is to understand what the disorder is and what to do to minimize and manage the symptoms. Hiding your head in the sand and pretending that ADHD is not there will not improve your self-esteem.

Think of it this way: the world is going to communicate to the individual with ADHD that they have problems. The question is, will that individual blame themselves and feel helpless and hopeless about changing those problems or will they see that they have a real disorder and learn that they can manage it effectively? Which of those paths do you think is more likely to cause damage to self-esteem?

There are two additional points that should be made here. First, it may be that the answer we offered above will not be the best answer if the young person has only very mild symptoms of ADHD. If they are not getting a negative message from the world and are not likely to face significant challenges at college, then a lighter approach might be appropriate.

But please be very careful with that last point. In most cases, we find that people jump at this option for the wrong reasons. They want to believe that ADHD is not a major issue for the given individual, when in fact it is a major issue. Often, trying to pretend the problem is smaller than it is ends up making it way bigger than it ever needed to be.

The second point that must be made is that a young person with ADHD needs accurate information about his disorder if focusing on the disorder is going to have a positive result. If the message is, in effect, "you have ADHD, so give up on having a good life," then yes, that message would impact his self-esteem and confidence negatively. But that message is a lie. He should be told something like "you have ADHD and, while you may wish you didn't have it at all, you definitely can learn about the disorder and learn ways of managing it, and if you do that you absolutely can have a wonderful life."

Question 25: What questions are not answered in this book?

As we said earlier, we want this Skinny Book™ to provide streamlined answers to the questions that people often have as well as answers to questions that they would have if they knew more about the topic. That streamlined approach has its advantages, but now that you have an introduction to the topic, you may want a more comprehensive discussion of these issues.

That's why we are planning a series of books to address this topic. This book has a more comprehensive companion book that addresses the challenges an ADHD student faces in finding an

ADHD friendly college, applying to colleges, and preparing for college by making plans, learning coping skills, and preparing tools and resources during the senior year of high school.

This more comprehensive book is available now, either for sale or for preorder. We hope, in the near future, to also offer an additional pair of books, including one Skinny Book™ and one more comprehensive book, specifically addressing ways of setting the ADHD student up for success during the first year of college.

We hope that this Skinny Book™ and all the other books in the series will provide wonderful tools and information for all of the college bound ADHD students out there as well as all the adults that want to support an ADHD student and encourage their college success.

Other Books Coming Soon!

What if it's Time to go to college and my child has ADHD: Seven steps to creating a successful transition for college bound ADHD students

In this book, Drs. Paul and Kerri Nevin provide a clear blueprint for setting college bound ADHD students up for real and lasting success. This guide is designed to be the definitive "streetwise" handbook for college bound ADHD students themselves and also, particularly, for the adults who wish to provide support and guidance to such students. Parents overwhelmed by the prospect of sending an ADHD child to college, as well as counselors, therapists, coaches and college advisors will all find this book to be an invaluable resource.

Seven steps are outlined that will facilitate the transition to college. From providing information about finding an ADHD friendly college, to engaging a young person with ADHD in discussion about ADHD, to understanding medication options relevant to the college lifestyle, to a crash course in technology that might help support the ADHD student, all of the most important bases are covered in order to prepare an ADHD student to thrive during their college years.

This a book that strives to provide just the right amount of information, not too much or too little, so as to provide a one-stop resource for all those who feel overwhelmed by the prospect of helping a college bound ADHD student prepare for the college transition.

Resources

Barkley, R.A., Murphy, K.R., and Fischer M. (2008) ADHD in Adults: What the science says. New York, Guilford Press.

Barkley, R.A. (2010) Taking Charge of Adult ADHD. New York, Guilford Press.

Gordon, M. and McClure, F.D. (2008) The Down and Dirty Guide to Adult ADHD (2nd Ed.) DeWitt NY: GSI Publications.

Grossberg, B. (2011) Applying to College for Students with LD or ADD: A guide to keep you (and your parents) sane, satisfied, and organized through the admission process. Washington DC: Magination Press.

Kravets, M. and Wax, I.F. (2010) The K & W Guide to College for Students with Learning Disabilities or Attention Deficit Hyperactivity Disorder (ADHD) (10th Ed.): A resource book for students, parents, and professionals.

Maitland, T. L. and Quinn, P. (2011) Ready for Take-Off: Preparing your teen with ADHD or LD for college. Washington DC: Magination Press.

Nadeau K.G. (1994) Survival Guide for College Students with ADD or LD. Washington DC: Magination Press.

Quinn, P. (2012) AD/HD and the College Student: The everything guide to your most urgent questions. Washington DC: Magination Press.

Quinn, P. and Maitland, T. L. (2011) On Your Own: A college readiness guide for teens with ADHD/LD. Washington DC: Magination Press.

Peterson's Colleges for Students with Learning Disabilities or ADHD. (8th Edition.)

Sandler, M. (2008) College Confidence with ADD. Naperville IL: Sourcebooks Inc.

Sarkis, S. (2008) Making the Grade with A+DD: A students guide to succeeding in college with attention deficit disorder. Oakland, CA: New Harbinger Publications Inc.

Tuckman, A. (2009) More Attention, Less Deficit: Success strategies for adults with ADHD. Plantation FL: Specialty Press.

Websites

www.addconsults.com

This site describes itself as "Helping women with ADD get unstuck and ontrack" and "The place to find ADD resources, professionals, consulting services and products.

www.add.org

A non-profit organization providing help to adults with ADHD.

www.ADDitudemag.com

A variety of resources for adults with ADHD including articles and printable resources, as well as connections to blogs, coaches, groups and more.

www.Chadd.org

For those not familiar with CHADD, it is the "Children and Adults with Attention Deficit Disorder" support organization. They offer comprehensive advice and resources for individuals and families dealing with ADHD.

www.RussellBarkley.org

A very valuable site with ADHD fact sheets, courses, links to other resources, and many other things. Barkley provides a "Consensus statement on ADHD," signed by numerous professionals in the field, which goes a long way toward showing that most of the debate about the validity of ADHD is fictional, at least among health and mental health professionals. You can also find some wonderful summaries regarding adult ADHD from Dr. Barkley on YouTube.

www.totallyadd.com

The makers of the film "ADD and loving it," about a comedian diagnosed with ADHD written by another comedian with ADHD. Light hearted presentation of serious information about ADHD, including material related to adult ADHD.

www.transition2college.com

An excellent site not only for ADHD students, but for all students with disabilities going to college.

www.ingramcontent.com/pod-product-compliance
Lightning Source LLC
Chambersburg PA
CBHW061300040426
42444CB00010B/2434